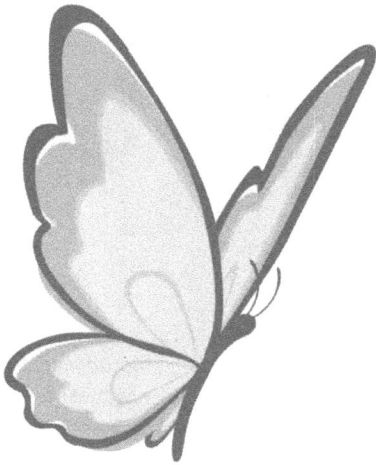

Symptom Free

From:

"Irritable Bowels"

Identifying the triggers that
influence bowel symptoms, such as bloating and diarrhoea

Including everything you need to know for
achieving a low FODMAP diet

Suitable for people with IBS or fructose malabsorption

Symptom Free From: Irritable Bowels

Author: Kerry Withoos

Copyright @ 2013

Updated 2014

National Library of Australia Cataloguing-in-Publication entry

Author:	Withoos, Kerry.
Title:	Symptom free from irritable bowels
ISBN:	9780646563961 (pbk.)
Subjects:	Malabsorption syndromes – Diet therapy – Recipes. Food allergy – Diet therapy. Irritable Colon – Diet therapy – Recipes. Health.
Dewey Number:	613

Published with the assistance of:

www.loveofbooks.com.au

Introduction

This book is written for anyone wishing to be free from symptoms of 'Irritable Bowels'.

If you have been diagnosed with Irritable Bowel Syndrome or fructose malabsorption, or if you suffer with one, or more, of the following symptoms: bloating, wind, cramping, nausea, diarrhoea and/or constipation, then this book is written for you.

Years of research and practical experience with hundreds of clients, has resulted in identifying the specific dietary and lifestyle triggers that have the greatest influence on Irritable Bowels. I discuss each of these triggers in great detail and I explain how you can identify the triggers that influence your bowels. I provide detailed lists of foods to choose and foods to avoid, including an entire chapter on the FODMAP carbohydrates, detailed shopping guides, strategies for dining out, sample meal and snack plans, healthy eating tips, label reading information, recipes and more.

I look forward towards assisting you on your journey to becoming symptom free from Irritable Bowels.

Kerry Withoos

Kerry Withoos

Accredited Practising Dietitian, Accredited Nutritionist

Contents

Getting Started

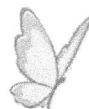

1

I am very pleased to be assisting you on your journey towards becoming symptom free from Irritable Bowels.

For the purposes of this book, I define 'Irritable Bowels' as having been diagnosed with Irritable Bowel Syndrome or fructose malabsorption or having one, or more, of the following symptoms: bloating, wind, cramping, nausea, diarrhoea and/or constipation. These symptoms can not only be embarrassing, but they can be quite distressing and may have an impact on your quality of life.

As a professional dietitian specialising in bowel issues for many years, I have seen hundreds of clients with symptoms of Irritable Bowels. These clients are now successfully managing their symptoms by having learnt to identify the dietary triggers that influence their bowels.

Throughout my teenage and early adulthood years I too suffered with Irritable Bowels, diagnosed as Irritable Bowel Syndrome. My symptoms included bloating, wind and diarrhoea. After years of research I was able to identify the specific triggers that influence Irritable Bowels. By minimising the triggers that influence my bowels I continue to remain symptom free. I now wish to assist you on your journey to becoming symptom free.

Because everybody is an individual, particularly where the bowels are concerned, learning how to manipulate your diet specifically for you is an important strategy for becoming symptom free. You may have spent years trying many different methods to resolve your symptoms, however typically it is not until all of the dietary and lifestyle triggers that influence your bowels are minimised that symptom relief is achieved.

The most effective approach for working with the information in this book is to commence by minimising all of the Irritable Bowel triggers that I discuss. The majority of you will notice a significant difference within several days. It is important to understand that this is not a long term diet plan. It is designed to help you discover which triggers are causing your symptoms and which triggers are not. After approximately 6 to 8 weeks of minimising all of the triggers you can then commence the next phase, which I have called the 'Challenge Phase'. The Challenge Phase is designed to determine which triggers influence your symptoms and which do not.

The triggers that have the greatest influence on Irritable Bowels are discussed in detail in the following chapters. These include: FODMAP carbohydrates, stress, fat, fibre, probiotics, meal size, fluid intake, caffeine, spicy foods, alcohol, artificial sweeteners, gas and exercise.

In some people, these Irritable Bowel triggers can exert an additive effect, i.e. one or two triggers may be well tolerated, however symptoms can occur if more triggers are included in one meal or in one day.

Chapter 2 begins with an explanation of the FODMAP carbohydrates. The majority of my clients experience the greatest relief by minimising the FODMAP carbohydrates.

Chapter 3 covers the other Irritable Bowel triggers in detail. Further chapters cover strategies for achieving a healthy, nutritionally balanced diet whilst minimising the triggers, including tips for creating a healthy eating plan, meal and snack ideas, detailed shopping lists, label reading and strategies for dining out. Chapter 9 explains the Challenge Phase which is designed to identify the triggers that cause your symptoms. The final chapter contains many easy to prepare, nutritious, Irritable Bowel trigger free recipes.

Before making any changes to your diet, it is <u>very</u> important that you have investigated other potential causes for your symptoms, such as Coeliac Disease, Inflammatory Bowel Disease, ovarian cancer and so forth. It is important that you do not self diagnose any bowel symptom. If your health professionals have found no apparent cause for your symptoms, or if you have been diagnosed with Irritable Bowel Syndrome or fructose malabsorption, then please read on because reducing the Irritable Bowel triggers in your diet should have you symptom free in no time at all.

Good luck on beginning your journey. I do appreciate your feedback and would encourage you to write to me with any comments that you may have. Contact details are provided at the end of the book.

The FODMAPs

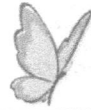

FODMAP carbohydrates may not be as well tolerated as other carbohydrates in people with Irritable Bowels. Once these FODMAP carbohydrates are consumed it appears they are not absorbed by the small intestine as well as they should be and subsequently travel to the large bowel where bacteria ferment them producing gas. Water is additionally drawn into the bowels and it is this gas and fluid that can produce symptoms such as bloating, wind, cramping and diarrhoea.

Some people with Irritable Bowels may experience constipation from consuming a diet higher in FODMAP carbohydrates. Recent research suggests that this may be because a different type of gas is produced by the bacteria during the fermentation process which can slow down bowel transit, resulting in constipation.

The research team at Monash University Eastern Health Clinical School in Australia have been the leading researchers into these fermentable carbohydrates and developed the term, FODMAPs, to encompass all of these fermentable molecules.

FODMAPs is an acronym for:

Fermentable
Oligosaccharides
Disaccharides
Monosaccharides

And

Polyols

Fermentable refers to these molecules being fermented by bacteria in the large intestine. Our intestines are a host for billions of bacteria that feed on substrates in the intestines which is a normal part of the digestive process. In people with Irritable Bowels this process can be exaggerated, therefore resulting in symptoms.

Oligosaccharides refers to molecules that include fructans and galacto-oligosaccharides (GOS). Examples of foods that contain fructans and GOS are wheat and chickpeas.

Disaccharides include the molecule lactose. This is the type of sugar found in milk and milk products including cow's milk and ice-cream.

Monosaccharides refers to fructose. Examples of foods that contain fructose include honey and mangoes.

Polyols includes sugar alcohols such as sorbitol and mannitol. These can be found in 'sugar free' products, including sugar free gum and sugar free mints. Sugar alcohols are also found naturally in some foods such as apricots and mushrooms.

The following table lists foods that contain FODMAP carbohydrates which was correct at the time of publishing. As this is a relatively new field of science, data is constantly changing so please be sure to visit my website for updates: www.irritablebowels.com.au.

In getting started on your journey towards identifying which triggers influence your bowels, it is a good idea to try and minimise as many FODMAP carbohydrates as possible. Whilst you may be able to tolerate small amounts of FODMAP carbohydrates at a time, they do have a cumulative effect in the bowels (the more you consume the greater chance you may get symptoms). For the initial 6 – 8 weeks, it is worthwhile minimising as many as you can.

In Chapter 9 we discuss strategies to determine your tolerance to FODMAP carbohydrates and the other Irritable Bowel triggers.

Table of foods containing FODMAPs and foods low in FODMAPs

Fruits

LOW FODMAP	CONTAIN FODMAPS
Banana	Apples
Blueberries	Apricots
Grapes	Avocado
Honeydew melon	Blackberries
Kiwi fruit	Cherries
Lemons	Custard apple
Lime	Dates
Mandarins	Dried fruit
Orange	Figs
Passionfruit	Fruit juice
Pawpaw	Guava
Pineapple	Longon
Raspberries	Lychee
Rhubarb	Mango
Strawberries	Nectarines
Tangelo	Peaches
	Pears

	Persimmon Plums Prunes Sugar bananas Tinned fruit (unless low FODMAP fruit in syrup) Water melon

Vegetables

LOW FODMAP	CONTAIN FODMAPS
Alfalfa	Artichoke
Bamboo shoots	Asparagus
Beans, green	Beetroot
Bean sprouts	Broccoli
Bok choy	Brussels sprouts
Capsicum	Butternut pumpkin
Carrot	Cabbage
Chives	Cauliflower
Cucumber	Celery
Eggplant	Chicory
Lettuce	Fennel
Olives	Garlic
Parsnip	Gherkin
Potatoes	Leek
Pumpkin (not butternut)	Legumes (chickpeas, lentils, kidney beans etc.)
Silverbeet	Mushrooms
Spinach	Onion – in all forms
Spring onion (green part only)	Peas
Swede	Radish
Tomato	Snow peas
Turnip	Squash
Yams	Sugar snap peas
Zucchini	Sweet corn
Watercress	Sweet potato
Water chestnut	Tomato products in concentrated forms (including tomato paste and tomato juice)

Breads / Grains

LOW FODMAP	CONTAIN FODMAPS
Amaranth	Barley
Arrowroot	Rye
Buckwheat	Semolina
Gluten free breads, rolls, pita breads, pizza bases	Wheat and wheat derivatives including: bulgur, couscous, durum, kamut, spelt
Gluten free rice cakes, corn cakes, crisp breads	Wheat products such as breads, pastas, biscuits, crackers, cakes, pizza bases, pita breads
Gluten free flours	
Gluten free pasta	
Maize (corn)	
Millet	
Oats	
Polenta	
Quinoa	
Rice	
Rice noodles	
Sago	
Sorghum	
Tapioca	

Dairy

LOW FODMAP	CONTAIN FODMAPS
Butter and margarine	Butter milk
Cheese – hard cheese such as cheddar cheese, parmesan cheese, tasty cheese	Cheese – processed, including cheese singles
Lactose free milk	Cheese – soft
Liddells™ Lactose Free Yoghurt	Condensed milk
Rice milk	Custard
	Evaporated milk
	Ice cream
	Milk, including cow, goat and sheep milk
	Yoghurt

Miscellaneous

LOW FODMAP	CONTAIN FODMAPS
	LEGUMES Beans (baked beans, borlotti,etc) Chickpeas, lentils
SAUCES/DRESSINGS Lemon juice Lime juice Wheat free soy sauce	**SAUCES/DRESSINGS** BBQ sauce Chutneys Curry / coconut sauces Fruit pastes Plum sauce Relish Sweet and Sour sauce
DRINKS Espresso coffee Black tea Green tea White tea Peppermint tea Dry red wine Dry white wine Spirits Mineral water (plain) Soda water (plain)	**DRINKS** Instant coffee Chicory based coffee substitutes Cocoa Drinking chocolate Carob powder Chamomile tea Infused herbal teas Infused fruit teas Oolong tea Chai tea Fennel tea Dandelion tea Fruit juice
SWEETENERS Aspartame, saccharine, stevia, sugar, glucose, glucose syrup	Port Sherry Sweet wine Champagne Rum

SPREADS	SWEETENERS
Freedom Foods™ Vege Spread	Sorbitol, mannitol, xylitol,
Glucose syrup	isomalt
Strawberry jam [check labels]	
Marmalade [check labels]	
Peanut butter	**SPREADS**
Rice syrup	Honey
Pure maple syrup	Soybean paste
	Agave syrup
NUTS/SEEDS	
Nuts not containing fodmaps	
*Limit nuts to two Tbsp per	
serve	**NUTS/SEEDS**
Seeds	Almonds
	Hazelnuts
	Cashews
	Pistachio nuts
	MISCELLANEOUS
	Agave syrup
	Inulin
	Chocolate toppings
	Coconut milk and cream
	Diet products including sugar
	free gum, diet jellies, sugar free
	mints
	Fruit flavoured toppings
	Liquorice

Note:
Some foods listed in the 'Contains FODMAPs' table above are lower in FODMAPs and are usually tolerated in smaller serves. These include:

Avocado (< ¼ cup per serving)
Beetroot (4 slices per serving)
Broccoli (< ½ cup per serving)
Butternut pumpkin (< ½ cup per serving)

Corn (< ½ cob per serving)
Fennel (< ½ cup per serving)
Peas (< ⅓ cup per serving)
Sweet potato (< ½ cup per serving)

The Other Irritable Bowel Triggers   3

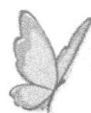

FODMAP carbohydrates are not the only triggers that can cause symptoms in people with Irritable Bowels. Other triggers include stress, fat, fibre, probiotics, meal size, fluid intake, caffeine, spicy foods, alcohol, artificial sweeteners, gas and exercise. Until your Challenge Phase, aim to minimise as many of the following Irritable Bowel triggers as possible.

Stress

Stress can play a significant role in people with Irritable Bowels. Increased levels of stress can stimulate bowel spasms which can lead to cramping and diarrhoea. The gastrointestinal system has many nerves that travel to the brain (called the gut-brain axis) and when a person is under stress, the bowels can respond. You may have experienced this in other ways such as nervous 'butterflies' prior to an important event.

When stress levels are high many people with Irritable Bowels will experience symptoms despite controlling for dietary triggers. Worrying about symptoms creates a vicious cycle: as stress levels increase, so too do bowel symptoms, leading to additional stress. If symptoms are brought on by increased stress levels, controlling or reducing these stressors will make a significant difference. Try as many different stress reducing strategies as possible until you find one that works for you. Studies have demonstrated that counselling, therapy and hypnotherapy are effective strategies for assisting with the stress related symptoms of Irritable Bowel

Syndrome and these may be well worthwhile investigating. Exercise is a great stress reliever and the additional benefits of exercise on Irritable Bowels are discussed below.

Diet

Diet can have a tremendous influence on the bowels. We have covered the FODMAPs in Chapter 2 and here we will cover other dietary triggers that can influence Irritable Bowels. As with the FODMAP carbohydrates, the triggers identified below can exert a cumulative effect, therefore try and minimise as many triggers as you can until the Challenge Phase, where we determine the triggers that influence your bowels.

Fat

High fat meals or snacks can cause painful cramping and loose stools in many people with Irritable Bowels. This is because too much fat at one time can stimulate the bowels to contract and subsequently increase the transit time of bowel motions. Maintaining a low fat diet can assist in the management of bowel symptoms and will have additional benefits for your overall health and well-being. Choosing low fat products, such as low fat, lactose free milk, low fat cheese and lean cuts of meat, as well as minimising fats and oils in cooking, are important steps towards achieving a low fat diet.

Here are some further strategies to help ensure that you are consuming a low fat diet:

- Where possible, read fool labels and aim to choose foods that contain less than 10g of fat, ideally less than 3g of fat, per 100g serve.

- Look for products that are labelled 'low fat' or 'skim', particularly dairy products.

- Avoid fatty meats, such as sausages and salami, and purchase lean cuts of meat with little, if any, visible fat.

- Trim all fat from meats before cooking and remove skin from poultry.

- Use oil sprays and non-stick pans for cooking.

Fibre

It is worthwhile assessing your tolerance to fibre. In many people with Irritable Bowels a particularly high fibre diet can aggravate symptoms, whereas in others, particularly those with constipation, insufficient fibre can exacerbate symptoms.

Fibre is the indigestible part of plants found in cereals, fruits and vegetables. Fibre is a significant component of a healthy diet and it is necessary for keeping bowel contents moving through the intestines.

Just as the _amount_ of fibre can play a role in people with Irritable Bowels, so too can the _type_ of fibre.

There are two major types of fibre: soluble fibre and insoluble fibre. Many people with Irritable Bowels find that gradually increasing soluble fibre is most beneficial for them, whereas others, particularly those with constipation, achieve the most benefit from the bulking effects of gradual increases in insoluble fibre. When making changes to your fibre intake it is important to increase amounts gradually to allow time for your bowels to adapt. It is equally as important to ensure an adequate fluid intake (see below).

Types of fibre:

Whilst most foods contain a combination of both types of fibre, some foods are higher in one type and therefore provide a good source for that type of fibre.

<u>Soluble fibre</u>

Soluble fibre forms a gel with water in the digestive tract and can slow down the digestive process. Overall, soluble fibre appears to be better tolerated in people with Irritable Bowels, particularly so for those with diarrhoea.

- **Low FODMAP Sources of Soluble Fibre:** Peeled fruits (for example, oranges, bananas, strawberries) and peeled vegetables (for example, potatoes, pumpkin), rice, gluten free pasta, oats, oat bran, flaxseed.

Insoluble fibre

Insoluble fibre does not dissolve in water and adds bulk to bowel motions. This helps stools move through the intestines, reducing the risk of constipation. Insoluble fibre tends to speed up the digestive process.

- **Low FODMAP Sources of Insoluble Fibre:** Wholegrain, gluten free cereal products, skins on fruit and vegetables.

Tips to ensure an adequate (low FODMAP) fibre intake:

- Aim for at least 2 servings of fruit throughout the day. For example, an orange with lunch and a cup of strawberries with afternoon tea.

- Include salad / vegetables at least twice a day. For example, sliced tomato, cucumber, lettuce and grated carrot in a sandwich for lunch and cooked vegetables served with dinner.

- Choose whole grains where possible. Suitable, low FODMAP whole grains include: brown rice, wild rice, buckwheat, amaranth, millet, quinoa and sorghum.

- Choose wholegrain or multigrain gluten free breads and crackers as well as wholegrain, or fibre enriched, gluten free pastas such as Orgran™ Essential Fibre pasta range.

- Add oat bran, rice bran or flaxseeds to breakfast cereals and smoothies.

- Include 2 tablespoons of nuts or seeds with meals and snacks.

Overall, it is important to assess your individual tolerance to fibre. If you are prone to diarrhoea trial increasing small amounts of soluble fibre, slowly and with ample water. For constipation, it may be worthwhile trialling gradual increases in insoluble fibre, again slowly and with ample water.

Probiotics

Normal, healthy bowels are inhabited with millions of good and bad bacteria, consisting of approximately 400 different strains. A contributing factor in Irritable Bowel symptoms appears to be the balance between this good and bad bacteria.

Supplementing with a daily probiotic may help restore the good bacteria in the bowels therefore relieving symptoms in some people. However, it is worth noting that not everyone benefits from supplementing with probiotics and some may experience an increase in symptoms, particularly bloating and wind.

Of the many studies evaluating the effects of probiotics on Irritable Bowel Syndrome, the probiotic strain Bifidobacteria has shown the most promising benefits for alleviating symptoms. If you do experience additional bloating or wind when trialling a probiotic do persist for several weeks to allow your bowels the time to adapt.

Regular meals and snacks

Consuming a regular meal and snack pattern of three small meals and two to three healthy snacks is a good principle for people with Irritable Bowels. Large, heavy meals can be difficult to digest and can put extra load on your digestive system, which may lead to symptoms. A well-balanced meal and snack regime, of appropriate portion sizes, may assist with symptom control. See the menu planning chapter for further ideas on appropriate portion sizes for both meals and snacks. As a general guide, aim to keep your dinner portions to these amounts:

- Carbohydrates (including potato, rice, pasta or corn) should resemble the size of your fist, or no more than a quarter of your dinner plate.
- Protein (such as meat, chicken or fish) should be the size of the palm of your hand, or no more than a quarter of your dinner plate.
- Fill the remaining half of your plate with low FODMAP salad / vegetables.

Adequate Fluid

An insufficient fluid intake can contribute to constipation. Dry, hard stools which are difficult to pass can irritate the lining of the bowels further increasing the risk of symptoms.

An adequate fluid intake is an important step towards alleviating constipation. If you are more prone to diarrhoea, it is equally important to ensure an adequate fluid intake due to the amount of fluid lost in your bowel motions.

In addition, fibre requires sufficient fluid to be effective and ensuring an adequate fluid intake will enable this process to occur efficiently.

Aim for around 6 to 8 cups of fluid (preferably water) each day.

Caffeine

Caffeine, found predominately in coffee, tea, cola drinks, energy drinks and chocolate, stimulates bowel contractions which can lead to cramping and/or diarrhoea in many people with Irritable Bowels. Instant coffee has recently been found to contain fodmaps. Espresso coffee is a better option.

If you experience cramping and/or diarrhoea, it may be worthwhile minimising caffeine to assess if caffeine is a trigger for you.

Spicy Foods

As with caffeine, spicy foods can stimulate the bowels to contract, which may lead to cramping and/or diarrhoea. If spicy foods such as chilli, peppers, jalapenos, Cajun foods, turmeric, cayenne pepper, curry and so forth cause symptoms, then these are best minimised.

Alcohol

Alcohol is another bowel stimulant that you will need to assess your tolerance levels to. Many people with Irritable Bowels find that all forms of alcohol need to be avoided, whilst others find that a small glass of dry red wine, for example, will not evoke symptoms.

Artificial Sweeteners

Artificial sweeteners may cause symptoms even in people without Irritable Bowels. It is best to try and avoid products that contain artificial sweeteners, including artificially sweetened drinks, gums, mints and lollies.

Gas

Most people with Irritable Bowels have enough gas in their intestines already causing symptoms such as wind and bloating. Chewing gum, drinking through straws and consuming carbonated drinks can all contribute to additional gas in the gastrointestinal tract and reducing these may help alleviate symptoms.

Exercise

Regular exercise is not only beneficial for your bowels, but has numerous benefits for your health and well being. Keeping as active as possible, with a daily walking regime for example, will help to keep your digestion system running optimally, assist with alleviating wind and easing bloating and constipation. Additionally, establishing a regular exercise regime will help to manage stress levels (a major Irritable Bowel trigger).

Creating Your
Healthy Eating Plan 4

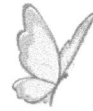

Achieving a nutritious, well-balanced, healthy diet is important for maintaining good health and well-being. As you will be minimising certain foods it, is necessary that you are replacing these with their nutritional equivalent.

Although it is quite easy consuming a healthy diet whilst minimising the Irritable Bowel triggers, it does take some thought and planning. At least for the first few weeks, it is worthwhile planning your meals and snacks in advance. This will help to ensure that you are not missing out on any of the important food groups.

What to aim for each day:

To ensure a nutritionally complete diet, aim to achieve the following number of serves from each of the food groups on a daily basis.

Fruits

2 to 3 serves of low FODMAP fruits

Keep serving sizes small. Large portions of even the allowed fruits may cause symptoms. As an example, add strawberries to your breakfast cereal in the morning and have an orange with lunch.

Vegetables

At least 5 serves of low FODMAP vegetables

To ensure adequate vegetables each day, aim to consume a serve of vegetables / salad at both lunch and dinner. Look for different coloured vegetables because each of the colours provides different beneficial nutrients. For example, add lettuce, tomato, grated carrot and cucumber to your sandwich at lunch and choose potato, pumpkin, green beans, carrot and spinach with dinner.

Dairy

At least 2 to 3 serves of calcium fortified, lactose free dairy foods

Dairy products provide important nutrients, including calcium. Ensure that your lactose free dairy products are calcium fortified and look for low fat or skim products where possible.

One serve of lactose free dairy equals:

- 30 – 40g of cheese (Bega™ So Extra Light 50% reduced fat cheese is a low fat, lactose free cheese)
- 250g of calcium fortified, low fat, lactose free milk
- 250g of calcium fortified rice milk (naturally low fat)
- 200g tub Liddells™ Plain, Lactose Free Yoghurt

If you are not consuming at least 2 to 3 serves of dairy products daily then it is important to ensure that you are consuming other calcium rich foods. The following list contains low FODMAP, dairy alternatives that contain calcium. Canned sardines, canned salmon with bones, ocean perch, trout, rhubarb, Bok Choy, spinach, tahini, oranges, sesame seeds, Brazil nuts, calcium fortified breakfast cereals (low FODMAP of course) and calcium fortified rice milk.

Breads and Cereals

<u>Include a serve at every meal (breakfast, lunch and dinner)</u>

The breads and cereals food group is important because it provides your body with fuel for energy as well as many nutrients, including dietary fibre. This food group should form the bulk of your dietary intake. Aim to include a serve at breakfast, lunch and dinner and choose whole grains where possible (see fibre section)

<u>Examples of this food group include:</u>

- Gluten free breads, gluten free pita breads, gluten free wraps, gluten free pizza bases and so forth.

- Low FODMAP breakfast cereals and porridges, including oat porridge, rice porridge, quinoa porridge, amaranth porridge.

- Wheat free biscuits and crisp-breads, including rice, oat and corn based

- Gluten free pasta and rice noodles

- Grains such as rice, quinoa, millet, amaranth, buckwheat, corn (maize), sago, polenta, sorghum

Protein

1 to 2 serves

Protein foods include:

- Meat

- Poultry (chicken and turkey)

- Fish

- Eggs

- Tofu

- Nuts and seeds

Protein foods do not typically irritate Irritable Bowels. Choose low fat protein foods by trimming fat from meats, removing skin from chicken and choosing small portions of nuts and / or seeds.

Sample Meals and Snacks 5

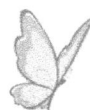

The key to optimum nutrition is choosing a wide variety of nutritious foods each day. Here is a range of ideas for both your meals and snacks to help ensure a wide variety.

Breakfast ideas

- Gluten free toast with vege spread, peanut butter, rice syrup, sliced banana or low fat cheese and tomato.
- Eggs (poached, boiled, scrambled or an omelette) with gluten free toast, tomato, capsicum and spinach.
- Oat porridge, quinoa porridge, amaranth porridge or rice porridge with allowed fruit or rice syrup to sweeten and topped with linseed meal, oat bran or rice bran for extra fibre.
- Low FODMAP breakfast cereal (for example: Freedom Foods™ Rice Puffs or Food for Health™ Clusters) with lactose free milk or rice milk, topped with fruit or rice syrup to sweeten and linseed meal, oat bran or rice bran for extra fibre.
- Fruit smoothie made using lactose free milk or rice milk, Liddells™ Lactose Free, Plain Yoghurt and fruit. Add linseed meal, oat bran or rice bran for extra fibre.
- Gluten free pancakes topped with lemon and sugar.
- Any recipe idea from the recipe section.

Lunch ideas:

- Sandwiches made with gluten-free bread. Add a protein, such as lean ham, chicken, turkey, tuna, salmon, sardines or egg and low FODMAP salad including, lettuce, tomato, cucumber and grated carrot.
- Eggs (poached, boiled, scrambled or an omelette) with gluten free toast and tomato, capsicum and spinach.
- Frittata with a side of low FODMAP salad vegetables.
- Low FODMAP salad bowl with boiled eggs, lean meat or tinned fish for protein and cooked, then cooled rice, gluten free pasta or potato for your carbohydrate portion.
- Baked potato topped with lean ham and low fat cheese, served with a low FODMAP salad.
- Rice paper rolls filled with low FODMAP vegetables including spinach, thinly cut sticks of carrots and capsicum and lean meat, chicken or fish.
- Sushi.
- Any breakfast or dinner idea.
- Any recipe idea from the recipe section.

Dinner ideas:

- Lean meat, chicken or fish served with potato and low FODMAP salad or vegetables.
- Gluten free pasta made with fresh tomatoes and lean mince meat, served with a low FODMAP salad. Use wheat free tamari sauce for flavour.

- Stir fry made with lean meat, chicken, fish or seafood, low FODMAP vegetables such as capsicum, carrot, water-chestnuts and bamboo shoots, using Tamari wheat free soy sauce mixed with rice syrup as a stir fry sauce. Serve with rice, rice noodles or gluten free pasta.

- Pizza made on a gluten free pizza base or gluten free pita bread, using low FODMAP vegetables such as tomatoes, pineapple, capsicum and spinach with ham and low fat cheese (avoid tomato paste and use fresh tomatoes on the pizza base instead).

- Rice paper rolls filled with lean meat, chicken or fish and low FODMAP vegetables.

- Savoury muffins (see recipe section) served with low FODMAP salad or vegetables.

- Tacos. Use corn taco shells and fill with lean mince meat, cooked in wheat free tamari sauce. Add to taco shells with chopped, low FODMAP salad vegetables including cucumber, capsicum, carrot and tomato and low fat cheese.

- Lasagne. Use gluten free lasagne sheets and layer with lean mince, low FODMAP vegetables and low fat cheese. For a white cheese sauce, mix a few tablespoons of corn flour with milk, over low heat, and stir in low fat cheese.

- Any lunch idea.

- Any recipe idea from the recipe section.

Desserts ideas:

- Fruit served with Liddells™ Lactose Free, Plain Yoghurt.
- Gelativo™ Fruit Sorbet.
- Homemade custard using gluten free custard powder and lactose free milk or rice milk.
- Rice cream or Sago (cooked with lactose free milk or rice milk) with fresh strawberries pureed or rice syrup to sweeten.
- Any snack idea.
- Any recipe idea from the recipe section.

Snack ideas:

Choose any of the following with a serving of low FODMAP fruit:

- Liddells™ Lactose Free, Plain Yoghurt.
- 2 tablespoons of nuts or seeds with an allowed fruit.
- Food for Health™ Fruit Free Muesli Bar.
- Rice or corn thins topped with tomato and low fat cheese.
- Fruit smoothie made with lactose free milk or rice milk, Liddells™ Lactose Free, Plain Yoghurt and fruit. Add linseed meal, oat bran or rice bran for extra fibre.
- Gluten free toast topped with tomato and low fat cheese.
- Packet Healtheries™ Rice Rounds or plain rice crackers.
- 20g plain potato chips.
- Low fat muffin (see recipe section).
- Any recipe idea from the recipe section.

Extra tips for flavouring:

Sauces and dressings can be high in FODMAPs and spices can be another potential trigger for Irritable Bowels, making it tricky adding flavour to foods. Here are some suggestions that may help:

- For a tasty marinade, salad dressing or stir fry sauce, mix equal amounts of wheat free soy sauce and rice syrup.
- Purchase garlic infused oil to help add flavour to your cooking.
- Try lemon juice and a touch of olive oil for salad dressings.
- Use small amounts of chives and the green part of spring onion in cooked dishes.
- Try asafoetida in cooking. Asafoetida is an Indian spice readily available in Indian shops. It has a strong onion-garlic flavour.

Trigger Free Shopping Guide

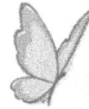

In this chapter I present tips and suggestions for purchasing low FODMAP, low trigger foods.

I have included a few examples for each of the food groups from my personal shopping list. This is not an exhaustive list by any means and there has been no intended inclusion or exclusion of any products at all.

There are countless of suitable products available. By following the tips suggested below and by reading ingredient lists, you will be able to stock up on a wide variety of products.

The examples provided are readily available at the major supermarket chains, typically in the health food section. You will notice that many (but not all) of the examples provided are labelled 'gluten free'. This is because 'gluten free' automatically excludes the FODMAP containing grains, wheat and rye. Unless you have Coeliac Disease, you should not have to follow a gluten free diet. Whilst 'gluten free' excludes wheat and rye, it does not exclude other FODMAP containing ingredients, so do check labels.

Shopping Guide

Breads / Cereals / Grains / Flours / Baking

Breads

Choose:

- 'Gluten free' breads to exclude wheat and rye.
- Wholegrain or multigrain where possible.

Examples:

- Country Life™ Gluten Free Multigrain or Low GI Bread
- Lifestyle Bakery™ Gluten Free Breads
- Burgen™ Gluten Free White Bread

Other Bread Products

Choose:

- Gluten free wraps, pita breads, bread mixes, pancake mixes and pizza bases.
- Wholegrain or multigrain where possible.
- Rice paper wraps and corn based taco shells.

Examples:

- Basco™ Bread Mix
- Orgran™ Buckwheat Pancake Mix
- Safeway™ Home-Brand Taco Shells
- True Foods™ Gluten Free Wraps
- Diego™ White Corn Tortillas
- Livwell™ Crumpets
- Livwell™ English Muffins

- Vitality™ Banana Bread
- Genius™ Gluten Free Pizza Base [freezer]

Breakfast cereals

Choose:

- Look for products labelled 'gluten free' and read ingredient labels to ensure that there is no added FODMAP carbohydrates such as dried fruit, fruit juice concentrate or honey.
- Consider making your own muesli. Look for suitable 'puffed' grains including buckwheat, rice, amaranth, quinoa and millet and mix equal parts. Add in a small portion of seeds or nuts as well as linseed meal, oat bran or rice bran for extra fibre.
- Porridges. Often sold as 'flakes' these are cooked in the same way as oat porridges. Look for oat porridge, rice porridge, quinoa porridge and amaranth porridge.

Examples:

- Food for Health™ Fruit Free Clusters and Fibre Cleanse Muesli
- Table of Plenty™ Nicely Nutty Muesli
- Freedom Foods™ Rice Puffs with Psyllium
- Kez's Free™ Low in Fructose Cereal
- Lowan™ Rice Flakes

Pasta / Noodles / Grains

Look for products labelled 'gluten free' and choose fibre enriched or wholegrain where possible.

Choose:

- Gluten free pasta, spaghetti, noodles and lasagne sheets.
- Rice noodles and rice vermicelli.
- Rice, including brown, white and wild rice.
- Quinoa, amaranth, millet, buckwheat, sago, tapioca, polenta, oats.

Examples:

- Changs™ Gluten Free Noodles
- Kan Tong™ Rice Noodles
- Orgran™ Essential Fibre Lasagnette
- Orgran™ Essential Fibre Rice and Corn Penne Pasta
- Orgran™ Supergrains Multigrain Pasta with Amaranth
- San Remo™ Gluten Free Macaroni
- San Remo™ Gluten Free Fettuccine

Flour / Baking Ingredients

Choose:

- Gluten free plain or self raising flour.
- Other suitable grain based flours including: rice flour, buckwheat flour, corn flour (maize flour), cornmeal, arrowroot flour, millet flour, potato flour and quinoa flour.
- Baking powder and baking soda.
- Glucose syrup, pure maple syrup and rice syrup.
- Aspartame, saccharine, stevia, sugar.

Snack Items

Muesli Bars

It can be difficult finding suitable muesli bars because many contain dried fruit and/or are sweetened with other FODMAP containing ingredients such as fruit juice, fruit juice concentrate, honey, fructose or high fructose corn syrup.

Choose:

- Bars that are sweetened with rice syrup or glucose syrup, both suitable ingredients.

Examples:

- Food for Health™ Gluten Free, Fruit Free Bar
- Kez's Free™ Gluten Free Cereal Snacks

Corn Cakes / Rice Cakes / Crispbreads

Choose:

- Corn, rice, millet, oat, quinoa, millet, buckwheat and other low FODMAP grain based cakes / thins / crisp-breads.
- Wholegrain or multigrain where possible.

Examples:

- Naturally Good™ Buckwheat Crispbread
- Orgran™ Essential Fibre Crispibread
- Orgran™ Toasted Multigrain Crispibread with Quinoa
- Real Foods™ Corn Thins Multigrain

Crackers / Savoury Biscuits

Read ingredient labels. Health food stores and the health aisles of supermarkets are good places to start.

Choose:

- 'Gluten free' biscuits (to exclude FODMAP containing grains) and check ingredients.

Examples:

- EsKal™ Deli Crackers (original)
- Eskal™ Pretzels
- Arnotts™ Corn Cruskits
- Healtheries™ KidsCare Rice Rounds
- Orgran™ Deli Crackers Multigrain with Poppyseed
- Orgran™ Gluten Free Supergrains Crispibread with Quinoa
- Spiral™ Tamari Rice Crackers

Chips / Crisps

Choose:

- Plain potato chips. Limit portions as chips are high in fat.
- Plain, air-popped popcorn.

Sweet Biscuits

Sweet biscuits are typically high in fat and therefore best kept to small portions occasionally.

Choose:

- 'Gluten free' biscuits (to exclude FODMAP containing grains) and check ingredients.

Examples:

- Butterfingers™ Shortbread
- Butterfingers™ Macadamia Shortbread
- Table of Plenty™ Dark Chocolate Mini Rice Cakes
- Eskal™ Tea Biscuits Vanilla
- Eskal™ Lemon Wafers
- Freedom Foods™ Gluten Free Triple Treat Brownie
- Freedom Foods™ Chocolate Blitz
- Kez's™ Free Melting Moments
- Orgran™ Outback Animals
- Orgran™ Shortbread Hearts

Cakes / muffins

Cakes and muffins are typically high in fat and therefore best kept to small portions occasionally.

Choose:

- 'Gluten free' (to exclude FODMAP containing grains) and check ingredients.

Examples:

- Basco™ Golden Butter Cake Mix
- Orgran™ Gluten Free Vanilla Cake
- Orgran™ Lemon Poppyseed Mix
- Well and Good™ All Purpose Cake Mix
- Well and Good™ Muffin Mix
- Macro™ Gluten Free Donut Mix
- Macro™ Gluten Free Cupcake Mix

- Coles Simply Gluten Free™ Orange & Chia Cake Mix
- Coles Simply Gluten Free™ Vanilla Cup Cake Mix

Dairy / Desserts

Cheese

Choose:

- All varieties of hard cheese such as tasty or cheddar.
- Low fat.

Examples:

- Bega™ So Extra Light & Tasty 50% Reduced Fat Cheese

Milk

Choose:

- Calcium fortified, lactose free cow's milk or rice milk.

Examples:

- Liddells™ Lactose Free Low Fat or Skim Milk
- Zymill™ Lactose Free Low Fat or Skim Milk
- Vitasoy™ Rice Milk

Yoghurt

Many yoghurts, including lactose free, contain inulin and fructose added as sweeteners, both of which are high in FODMAPs.

Choose:

- Liddells™ Lactose Free, Plain Yoghurt

Cream

<u>Choose:</u>

- Liddells™ Lactose Free Light Cream (sold as a long life cream)

Eggs

<u>Choose:</u>

- All varieties of eggs, including chicken and duck eggs.

Margarine / Butter

Butter contains only trace amounts of lactose and is therefore suitable, however it is high in saturated fat so use sparingly.

Margarines are a better option as they contain less saturated fat than butter.

<u>Examples:</u>

- Meadow Lea™ Extra Light Margarine
- Flora Pro Active™ Ultra Light Margarine
- Nuttelex™ Lite

Desserts

Suitable low FODMAP dessert options are limited.

Consider making your own desserts from the recipes provided at the end of the book.

<u>Choose:</u>

- Fresh fruit and Liddells™ Lactose Free, Plain Yoghurt.
- Homemade desserts.

<u>Examples:</u>

- Gelativo™ Fruit Sorbet

- Liddells™ Lactose Free, Plain Yoghurt
- Peters™ Lactose Free Ice-cream
- So Good™ Vanilla or Chocolate Bliss Ice-cream
- Coles™ Bakery Mini Pavlova
- White Wings™ Gluten Free Custard Powder

Fruit / Vegetables

Use the FODMAP table presented in Chapter 2 to choose low FODMAP fruit and vegetables.

Canned fruits are typically preserved in pear juice (which is high in FODMAPs) and therefore should be avoided. Purchase low FODMAP fruit that has been canned in syrup.

Choose:

- Frozen or tinned, low FODMAP vegetables without added ingredients.
- Frozen, low FODMAP fruit without added ingredients.
- Tinned, low FODMAP fruit in syrup

Examples:

- Great Lakes™ Strawberries in Syrup
- Golden Circle™ Pineapple Pieces in Syrup
- Admiral™ Mandarins in Syrup
- Creative Gourmet™ Frozen Blueberries

Meat / Poultry / Fish / Eggs

Protein foods, including meats, poultry (chicken, turkey), fish, tins of plain tuna, salmon or sardines, shellfish, eggs, tofu and so forth, are all free of FODMAP carbohydrates and should not cause symptoms.

Choose:

- Low fat options.

Spreads / Stocks

Spreads

Aside from honey, which is high in FODMAPs, most spreads are suitable. For higher fat spreads, such as peanut butter, keep to small portions.

Examples:

- Kraft™ Vegemite
- Peanut butter
- Freedom Foods™ Vege Spread
- Rice syrup or rice malt syrup (a great alternative to honey)
- Pure Maple Syrup
- IXL™ Conserve Strawberry jam
- IXL™ Marmalade Breakfast in Glass

Stocks / Gravies

Ensure that stocks and gravies are free from onion and garlic powder.

Examples:

- Spiral Foods™ Wheat Free Tamari Sauce
- Masterfoods™ Mild English Mustard

- Masterfoods™ Dijonnaise
- Massel 7's™ Chicken Stock Cubes
- Massel 7's™ Beef Stock Cubes
- Continental™ Beef Style Stock Cubes
- Campbell's™ Real Stock Chicken Stock (liquid)
- Gravox™ Traditional Gravy (tin)
- Gravox™ Chicken Gravy (tin)
- Gravox™ Roast Meat Gravy (tin)

Label Reading 7

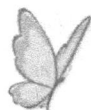

Understanding food labels will help you feeling confident that the products you are choosing are indeed low trigger foods. If the ingredient list is free of the triggers discussed in earlier chapters, as well as the ingredients presented below, then your product should be suitable.

What to look for on labels:

Sugar alcohols, including: sorbitol, mannitol, xylitol and isomalt, High fructose corn syrup, corn syrup solids, fructo-oligosaccharides, fructose, honey, fruit juice concentrate, inulin.

To maintain a low fat diet, where possible choose products that have less than 10g of fat (ideally less than 3g of fat) per 100g serve.

The following labels demonstrate ingredient lists that contain FODMAP carbohydrates (highlighted in bold):

Yoghurt
Ingredients: **Skim milk, Milk solids,** Fruit (orange, **apricot,** passionfruit), **Fructose,** Mineral salts, Gelatine, Natural colour, Live yoghurt cultures.

Muesli Bar
Ingredients: Peanuts, Almonds, **Dried apple, Dried apricot,** Sunflower seeds, Puffed **wheat, Honey,** Sunflower oil, Sugar, **Inulin,** Brown sugar, Emulsifier.

The following ingredient lists contain no FODMAP carbohydrates and are therefore suitable purchases.

Muesli Bar

Ingredients: Corn flakes, Rice bran syrup, Puffed rice, Puffed millet, Sorghum, Pepitas, Rice bran oil, Natural flavour

Crackers

Ingredients: Brown rice, wholegrain sorghum, wholegrain, millet, salt, poppy seed.

Oats Sachet

Ingredients: Wholegrain rolled oats, Brown sugar, Natural flavour

Tips & Strategies For Dining Out

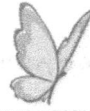

8

Dining out is certainly an enjoyable part of life. By scanning menus and choosing low FODMAP, low trigger options, you can continue to enjoy dining out, whilst ensuring that you remain symptom free.

Besides identifying potential trigger foods, other important factors to consider when dining out are large, over-sized portions and excess dietary fat. Both can irritate the bowels and both are common when dining out. Use the strategies provided below, such as choosing low fat options and ordering entree sized dishes rather than mains, to help keep your dining experiences Irritable Bowel trigger friendly.

General tips

- Consider restaurants that offer gluten free options. This way you are guaranteed a choice of wheat and rye free dishes that you can then modify to exclude other FODMAP ingredients and other potential triggers such as spices.

- Choose entree sized serves as your main to keep portions smaller. You can always add sides to your entree, including dressing free salads, steamed vegetables and steamed rice.

- Choose plain, grilled, lean meats, skinless chicken, fish or seafood without sauces, dressings or coatings.

- For the carbohydrate portion of meals, add a baked potato, a small serve of thickly cut chips (thicker chips contain less fat than thinner chips) or boiled rice.

- Order both a side of vegetables and a dressing free salad to provide more options to choose from.

Sauces and Dressings

- Avoid sauces and dressings as these may contain FODMAPs and are often high in fat.

Pasta

- Whilst you could choose a gluten free pasta if available, the accompanying sauce would most likely contain FODMAPs

Rice

Choose:

- Plain, boiled or steamed rice.

- Rice paper rolls with suitable fillings.

- Sushi.

Drinks

Choose:

- Plain water, mineral water or soda water (unless carbonated drinks cause symptoms). Add lemon or lime to flavour.

- If alcohol is not a trigger for you, choose the low FOMAP options such as dry red wine or spirits mixed with plain mineral or soda water. Add lemon or lime to flavour.

- Take your own milk for hot drinks.

Desserts

Choose:

- Order a fresh fruit salad and choose the low FODMAP fruits.

- Fresh strawberries sprinkled with icing sugar.

- Lemon gelato if available.

Dining at Friends' Homes

Many clients find dining at friends' or relatives' homes a little more challenging than dining out at restaurants because there is no menu to choose suitable dishes from.

A good strategy is to take a plate of low trigger food to share in order to provide at least one suitable option. See the recipe section for great tasting meal and dessert ideas.

Cafe

Choose:

- Sushi.

- Gluten free sandwiches if gluten free bread is available.

- Take your own gluten free bread and ask for a sandwich to be made with suitable ingredients.

- If gluten free bread is not available, ask for a salad plate to be made up of low FODMAP salads and include deli meats, eggs and/or fish for your protein serve.

Breakfast

Choose:

- Eggs (boiled or poached) with grilled tomato, lean bacon and gluten free toast if available.

- Take your own milk if porridge or gluten free cereals are available.

Asian

Choose:

- Boiled or steamed rice.

- Buckwheat noodles.

- Rice paper rolls with low FODMAP fillings.

- Plain, low FODMAP, stir fry vegetables with chicken, meat or seafood.

- Steamed fish.

Indian
Choose:

- Tandoori chicken or lamb.

- Steamed fish.

- Steamed or boiled rice.

- Plain, stir fry vegetable dishes.

Italian
Choose:

- Plain, grilled, lean meats, including veal and chicken.

- Seafood dishes such as steamed mussels.

- Low FODMAP, dressing and sauce free salads and vegetables.

Fish and Chips
Choose:

- Batter-free, grilled fish.

- Chips.

McDonalds™

Choose:

- Chicken or garden salads without the dressing.

- Fries.

- Hash browns.

Parties

Take a plate to share with others. Some ideas include:

- A platter of carrot, capsicum and cucumber sticks, hard cheese, nuts, rice crackers and home-made dip (cooked, mashed pumpkin works well as a dip).

- Fruit kebabs. Skewer segments of kiwi, mandarin, banana, pineapple, strawberries and orange.

- Top mini, gluten free pancakes with savoury toppings, such as smoked salmon.

- Cut gluten free wraps into triangles and bake for 10 minutes to create crispy, pita style chips.

It is unnecessary and too restrictive to eliminate all of the Irritable Bowel triggers long term. Many people find that they do not react to all of the triggers and of the ones that they may react to they are able to tolerate in small amounts. After approximately 6 to 8 weeks of minimising the Irritable Bowel triggers you can challenge yourself with each of the triggers to assess your tolerance levels.

A good way to approach this Challenge Phase is to commence with the FODMAP carbohydrates. The FODMAPs are classed into six groups (fructose, lactose, fructans, mannitol, sorbitol and galacto-oligosaccharides [GOS]) and I have presented a table below listing which foods fall into each of these six groups. You will find this table useful once you have determined which FODMAPs you react to and which FODMAPs you tolerate.

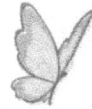

I have recommended the most suitable challenge food for each FODMAP group. Each of these foods contains just one FODMAP group. Many foods high in FODMAP carbohydrates contain more than one FODMAP group making them unsuitable for challenges. As an example, an apple contains both fructose and sorbitol and if you reacted to apple you would not be able to identify whether it was the fructose or the sorbitol causing the reaction.

It is best to challenge with just one FODMAP group each week, keeping the rest of the week's intake Irritable Bowel trigger free. Aim to have at least one Irritable Bowel trigger free day in between each challenge day to ensure no residual symptoms are being carried over into a subsequent challenge. It is also a good idea to test each FODMAP group at least twice. If you do experience symptoms after testing a FODMAP group twice then you can either: 1/ re-challenge with that group again, however this time halving the challenge amount or 2/ minimise that particular FODMAP group for a few more months and re-challenge again at a later date.

Once you have challenged a FODMAP group keep it out of your diet, even if you do not react to it, until you have finished challenging with all of the Irritable Bowel triggers.

As onion can be particularly problematic it is worthwhile testing this as a separate challenge.

FODMAP challenge foods:

Fructose

3 teaspoons of honey or 1 mango cheek.

Lactose

125mls of cow's milk or 200g of yoghurt. Many lactose containing yoghurts also contain fructose, therefore you will need to find a lactose containing, fructose free yoghurt for your challenge. Check labels of lactose containing yoghurts for ingredients such as inulin, fructose, honey, high FODMAP fruits and so forth.

Fructans

2 slices of wheat bread

Sorbitol

4 dried apricot halves or 2 fresh apricots

Mannitol

Half a cup of mushrooms or ⅓ cup cauliflower

Galacto-oligosaccharides

Half a cup of legumes (for example, cannelloni beans, lentils, chickpeas)

Getting Started:

Mannitol is one group that most of my clients seem to tolerate well, therefore this is a good FODMAP group to start with.

Some tips to remember:

1. Take at least a week to test each of the FODMAP groups, testing the same challenge food on two separate occasions, with at least one 'rest' day in between.
2. Ensure that your diet during this challenge period is free from all Irritable Bowel triggers, aside from the challenge food.
3. Remember to record any symptoms experienced.
4. If you do react to a FODMAP group then either:
    a. Retry that FODMAP group again in half the quantity
    b. Omit that group and rechallenge at a later date.

A Suggested Challenge Phase:

Be sure to record symptoms (if any) on all days.

Week 1 – Mannitol

Day 1:   Trial half a cup of mushrooms or ⅓ cup of cauliflower

Day 2:   Entire day is Irritable Bowel trigger friendly

Day 3:   Trial half a cup of mushrooms or ⅓ cup of cauliflower

Day 4:   Entire day is Irritable Bowel trigger friendly

Week 2 – Sorbitol

Day 1:   Trial 2 fresh apricots or 4 dried apricot halves

Day 2:   Entire day is Irritable Bowel trigger friendly

Day 3:   Trial 2 fresh apricots or 4 dried apricot halves

Day 4:   Entire day is Irritable Bowel trigger friendly

Week 3 – Fructans

Day 1:   Trial 2 slices of wholemeal bread

Day 2:   Entire day is Irritable Bowel trigger friendly

Day 3:   Trial 2 slices of wholemeal bread

Day 4:   Entire day is Irritable Bowel trigger friendly

Week 4 – Fructose

Day 1:   Trial half a mango cheek or 3 teaspoons of honey

Day 2:   Entire day is Irritable Bowel trigger friendly

Day 3:   Trial half a mango cheek or 3 teaspoons of honey

Day 4:   Entire day is Irritable Bowel trigger friendly

Week 5 – Lactose

Day 1:   Trial 125ml milk or 200g yoghurt

Day 2:   Entire day is Irritable Bowel trigger friendly

Day 3:   Trial 125ml milk or 200g yoghurt

Day 4:   Entire day is Irritable Bowel trigger friendly

Week 6 – Galacto-oligosaccharides

Day 1:   Trial ½ cup of legumes

Day 2:   Entire day is Irritable Bowel trigger friendly

Day 3:   Trial ½ cup of legumes

Day 4:   Entire day is Irritable Bowel trigger friendly

Week 7 – Onion

Day 1:   Trial ¼ cup of onion

Day 2:   Entire day is Irritable Bowel trigger friendly

Day 3:   Trial ¼ cup of onion

Day 4:   Entire day is Irritable Bowel trigger friendly

The following table lists the breakdown of the six FODMAP groups. Following your challenges, you can use this table to determine which foods you can include back into your diet and which foods you should minimise. As this is a relatively new science, information is continually being revised. Should any changes occur I will update these on my website: www.irritablebowels.com.au.

FODMAP breakdown

Please note that some foods contain more than one FODMAP and will therefore appear more than once.

Fructose	Apple	Asparagus	Artichoke
	Cherries	Dried fruit	Fruit juice
	High fructose corn	Honey	Mango
	syrup	Sugar snap	Tinned fruit in
	Pear	peas	natural juice
	Tomato paste	Watermelon	Wine

Fructans	Asparagus	Artichoke	Barley
	Beetroot	Broccoli	Brussels sprouts
	Butternut pumpkin	Chicory	Custard apple
	Dried fruit	Fennel	FOS*
	Garlic	Green peas	Inulin
	Leek	Nectarine	Okra
	Onion	Pistachio nuts	Peaches
	Persimmon	Rye	Snow peas
	Sweet corn	Watermelon	Wheat
Lactose	Buttermilk	Condensed milk	Custard
	Evaporated milk	Ice cream	Milk
	Soft cheese	Yoghurt	
Mannitol	Alcohol**	Cauliflower	Celery
	Mushroom	Peach (Clingstone)	Snow peas
	Sweet potato	Watermelon	
Sorbitol	Apricot	Apple	Avocado
	Blackberries	Cherries	Lychee
	Longon	Nectarines	Peaches
	Pears	Plums	Sugar free products
GOS	Brussels sprouts	Cabbage	Legumes (beans,
	Pistachio nuts		lentils, chickpeas)

*FOS: fructo-oligosaccharides

**Alcohol: Some wine and beer

Once you have tested each of the FODMAP groups and have identified the FODMAPs that you do and do not react to, you can then test the amounts of these foods that you tolerate. Just as everyone will react differently to each of the six FODMAP groups, the overall amount of FODMAPs tolerated is also very individual, making it difficult suggesting an appropriate 'one size fits all' challenge approach. It is therefore recommended that you adopt a 'trial and see' type method as you continue to increase your variety. For example, if the fructan and mannitol tests were tolerated you may next like to challenge with 2 slices of wholemeal bread for breakfast and include mushrooms for dinner on the same day.

Trialling foods that contain more than one FODMAP, such as an apple, is another challenge process as well as trialling the other Irritable Bowel triggers such as caffeine and spicy foods. As with testing the individual FODMAPs, start off with small amounts and work up (gradually) to your previous intake to determine your tolerance levels.

After completing the challenges you will be able to identify which triggers irritate your bowels and which triggers do not. It is my hope that by minimising the triggers that influence your bowels you will remain symptom free whilst continuing a healthy, nutritious and varied dietary intake.

I wish you all the very best.

Please feel free to contact me either through my website or by my email provided below.

For additional support, individual assistance, recipes, recipe photographs and updates please visit my website regularly: www.irritablebowels.com.au.   Email: kerry@irritablebowels.com.au

Recipes

I have created a number of Irritable Bowel friendly recipes that are simple and easy to cook and ones that your whole family and friends will be sure to love.

Most of these recipes are my own personal favourites. They use simple ingredients and are easy to prepare.

For large, colour photographs of each recipe below, please visit my website: www.irritablebowels.com.au

BREAKFAST RECIPES

Berry Bircher Muesli

Ingredients

- 4 tablespoons of Food For Health™ Clusters Muesli
- ⅓ cup of Liddells™ Lactose, Free Plain Yoghurt
- 2 tablespoons of blueberries
- 1 tablespoon of seeds

Method

Combine all ingredients, except for the seeds. Mix well, sprinkle with the seeds and serve. Serves 1

French Toast

Ingredients

- 2 eggs
- 2 teaspoons of caster sugar
- 140 ml lactose free milk or rice milk
- 4 slices of gluten free white bread
- Low fat margarine for frying
- Rice syrup to serve

Method

Lightly whisk the eggs in a bowl. Add the milk and sugar and stir to combine.

Melt low fat margarine in a large frying pan over medium to high heat. Soak the bread in the egg mixture and cook for 1 – 2 minutes each side until golden.

Serve with the rice syrup.

Serves 2

Mini Baked Eggs

Ingredients

- 3 slices of ham
- 2 eggs
- 2 tablespoons of low fat cheese, grated

Method

Preheat oven to 180°C. Lightly grease a ¾ cup capacity ovenproof dish and line with the ham, covering the base and sides.

Sprinkle the ham with the cheese and then crack the eggs into the dish.

Bake for around 15 to 20 minutes or until egg white is just set.

Remove from the oven and let stand for 2 minutes to completely set.

Serves 1

Rice Brekky

Ingredients

- ½ cup cooked rice
- 1 tablespoon linseeds
- 1 teaspoon chopped walnuts
- 1 teaspoon rice syrup
- ¼ cup lactose free milk or rice milk
- ½ teaspoon cinnamon

Method

Combine all ingredients, except the cinnamon, in a saucepan and warm over medium heat. Serve sprinkled with cinnamon.

Serves 1

BREADS / SAVOURY MUFFINS

Very Easy Cheesy Bread

Ingredients

- 1 ½ cups of gluten free self raising flour
- 1 tablespoon caster sugar
- 2 teaspoons baking powder
- ¾ cup polenta
- 1 cup low fat cheese, grated
- 2 tomatoes, one diced and one sliced
- 100g ham, chopped
- 2 eggs, lightly beaten
- 1 cup lactose free milk or rice milk
- ⅓ cup olive oil
- Salt and pepper to season

Method

Preheat oven to 180°C. Line a loaf tin with baking paper.

Mix the flour, sugar, baking powder, salt and pepper in a large bowl. Add the polenta, cheese, the diced tomato and ham.

In a separate bowl whisk the eggs, milk and oil and add to the flour mixture. Combine well. Add the mixture to the prepared loaf tin and top with the tomato slices. Bake for approximately 45 to 50 minutes, until a skewer comes out clean.

Mini Ham, Cheese and Tomato Muffins

Ingredients

- 1 medium potato, peeled
- 150g ham, diced
- 2 tomatoes, diced
- 6 eggs
- 1 ½ cups lactose free milk or rice milk
- ½ cup low fat cheese, grated + grated cheese for top

Method

Preheat oven to 180°C. Coat an 8 large (or 12 small) muffin tray with cooking spray.

Cook potato until tender and dice. Add the tomato and ham to the diced potatoes and fill each muffin cup half way with this mixture.

Combine the eggs and milk and pour into the muffin cups over the potato mixture. Sprinkle with cheese.

Bake larger muffins for 22 to 24 minutes or the smaller muffins for 18 to 20 minutes or until set and puffed up slightly.

Corn Muffins

Ingredients

- 1 cup polenta
- 2 eggs, lightly beaten
- 2 cups gluten free self raising flour
- 1 cup lactose free milk or rice milk
- 2 tablespoons oil
- 1 cup tinned corn, drained (note that 1 cup of corn over 12 muffins should be well tolerated, omit if overly sensitive)
- 1 cup low fat cheese, grated
- 1 cup low fat ham (optional)

Method

Preheat oven to 180°C. Grease a 12 capacity muffin tray.

Whisk the polenta and flour. Add the beaten egg, milk and oil. Add remaining ingredients and lightly mix.

Add mixture to muffin tray and bake for approximately 30 minutes.

ACCOMPANIMENTS / VEGETABLES / SALADS

Zucchini Fritters

Ingredients

- 2 zucchinis, grated
- ½ cup gluten free plain flour
- ¼ cup water
- 2 tablespoons parmesan cheese

Method

Combine all ingredients and mix well.

Using approximately 2 tablespoons of fritter, shape and cook in a non-stick pan, turning to brown both sides.

Polenta Squares

Ingredients

- 1 cup polenta
- 2 tablespoons low fat margarine
- ½ cup grated parmesan cheese
- 3 cups prepared, onion and garlic free, chicken stock

Method

In a saucepan bring the stock to the boil and stir in the polenta. Continue stirring until mixture is thick and creamy. Add the cheese and margarine and mix well.

Season and spoon polenta into a greased 20cm cake tin and refrigerate. When cold, cut into squares. Heat a non-stick pan and fry each side until crisp and golden.

Potato Bake

Ingredients

- 2 cups lactose free milk or rice milk
- ¼ cup Liddells™ Lactose Free, Light Cream
- ¼ cup low fat cheese, grated + extra for topping
- 5 medium potatoes, peeled and sliced thinly
- Salt and pepper to taste

Method

Preheat the oven to 180°C.

Combine the milk, cream and cheese in a saucepan, boil, remove from heat and season with the salt and pepper.

Place the potatoes in an oven proof dish and pour over the milk mixture. Cook uncovered for 1 hour, or until potatoes are soft. Top with the extra cheese and cook for a further 10 minutes, or until golden. Serves 6 as an accompaniment.

Roasted Pumpkin Salad with "Honey and Soy" Dressing

Ingredients

- 1 kg pumpkin (not butternut), cut into 2cm thick pieces
- ½ large cucumber, sliced
- 2 tomatoes, sliced
- ¼ cup walnuts, chopped
- Lettuce leaves and/or baby spinach
- ¼ cup rice syrup
- 2 tablespoons wheat free soy sauce

Method

Preheat the oven to 220°C and line a baking tray with baking paper.

Place the pumpkin in a single layer on the tray, spray with oil and roast for 20 minutes or until golden, turning once. Set aside to cool.

Combine the rice syrup and wheat free soy sauce in a screw-top glass jar and microwave (without the lid) for 10 seconds to melt the rice syrup. Secure lid and shake to combine.

Place the lettuce and/or baby spinach in a large salad bowl and add the cucumber, tomato, pumpkin and walnuts and drizzle with the dressing.

Serves 4 – 6

SOUPS

Chicken and Sweetcorn Soup

Ingredients

- 200g can creamed corn (note that 200g of corn in four servings should be well tolerated, omit if overly sensitive)
- 3 cups prepared, onion and garlic free, chicken stock
- 2 cups cooked chicken, roughly chopped (approximately 250g)
- 2 teaspoons wheat free tamari sauce
- 1 tablespoon rice syrup
- 1 teaspoon cornflour
- 2 egg whites, lightly beaten
- 2 tablespoons water

Method

Heat the chicken stock in a saucepan over medium heat. When simmering add the corn and cook for 5 minutes. Add the chicken, tamari and rice syrup and cook for a further 5 minutes. Make a paste with the cornflour and water and add to the soup, cooking for a further minute to thicken. Gradually stir in the egg white and stir through. Serve.

Serves 4

Carrot and Potato Soup with rice syrup

Ingredients

- 2 potatoes, peeled and quartered
- 6 carrots, halved
- 2 lots of ¼ cup rice syrup
- 2 teaspoons wheat free tamari sauce
- 2 tablespoons oil
- 1 litre prepared, onion and garlic free, chicken stock
- 500ml water

Method

Preheat the oven to 180°C and line a tray with baking paper. Toss the carrots, potatoes, oil and ¼ cup of rice syrup in a bowl, then place on the prepared tray and bake for approximately 40 minutes, or until soft and golden brown, turning occasionally.

When cool, add the 500ml of water and blend in a food processor until smooth. Transfer to a saucepan and add the stock, tamari and the remaining ¼ cup rice syrup and heat on medium heat for 5 minutes. Serves 4

LIGHT MEALS / LUNCH RECIPES

Cheese and Ham Rice Based Pie

Ingredients

- 3 cups cooked long grain rice
- 1 egg
- 2 tablespoon parmesan cheese, grated

Filling:

- 200g lean ham, diced
- 4 eggs, lightly beaten
- ½ cup Liddells™ Lactose Free, Light Cream
- 150g low fat cheese, grated
- Salt and pepper to season

Method

Pre-heat oven to 170°C. Grease a 23cm flan tin or quiche dish.
Combine the cooked rice, egg and the 2 tablespoons of parmesan
cheese in a bowl. Press into the prepared dish and bake for 15
minutes, or until just starting to turn golden brown.

To make the filling, mix the ham, egg, cream and cheese in a bowl
until well combined and season with salt and pepper. Pour into the
rice crust and bake for 15-20 minutes or until set and cooked
through.

Tuna and Vegetable Balls

Ingredients

- 1 cup cooked rice
- 60g low fat cheese, grated
- 185g can tuna, drained and flaked
- ½ cup carrot, grated
- ½ cup tomato, finely chopped
- 1 egg, lightly beaten
- 1 cup gluten free breadcrumbs
- Extra gluten free breadcrumbs to coat

Method

Preheat oven to 180°C and line a baking tray with baking paper. Combine all ingredients, except the extra breadcrumbs, and roll into small balls. Roll the balls in the extra breadcrumbs. Place on the prepared tray and bake for 20 minutes. Alternatively, gently fry until brown. Add toothpicks to serve. Can be served warm or cold.

Frittata

Ingredients

- 1 medium potato
- 1 capsicum
- 1 zucchini
- ¼ cup of low fat cheese, grated
- 5 eggs
- ½ cup lactose free milk or rice milk

Method

Preheat oven to 180°C. Lightly grease a 23cm pie dish.

Peel and dice the vegetables and arrange over the base of the pie dish. Combine the eggs, milk and cheese and pour over the vegetables. Bake for 40 minutes or until set.

Serves 4 to 6

Zucchini Slice

Ingredients

- 150g ham, diced
- 6 eggs
- ⅓ cup gluten free plain flour
- ⅓ cup lactose free milk or rice milk
- 2 zucchini's, grated with excess moisture squeezed out
- 1½ cups low fat cheese, grated

Method

Preheat oven to 180°C. Lightly grease a lamington tray.

Whisk the eggs and milk together. Stir in the zucchini, ham and cheese until well combined. Stir in the flour and add to the tray. Bake for 25 to 30 minutes or until golden brown.

MAIN MEALS

Chicken Oat Loaf

Ingredients

- 500g minced chicken breast
- 1 cup rolled oats or 1 cup rice flakes
- ¼ cup lactose free milk or rice milk
- 1 egg, lightly beaten
- 1 large carrot, grated
- 1 cup vegetables, chopped (for example, capsicum, zucchini)

Method

Preheat oven to 180°C.

Combine all ingredients and press into a loaf tin.

Bake for 45 – 50 minutes.

Easy Fish and Veggie Pie

Ingredients

- 400g can tuna, drained
- 1 cup corn kernels (note that one cup of corn in this recipe should be well tolerated, omit if overly sensitive)
- 1 small carrot, diced and cooked
- 1 small zucchini, diced and cooked
- 2 x 400g cans of chopped tomatoes, well drained
- Mashed potato (using 3 medium potatoes)

Method

Pre-heat oven to 180°C.

Place the tuna into a large ovenproof dish and top with the corn, then the vegetables and then the tomatoes. Cover with the mashed potatoes and spray with oil spray.

Bake for 25 minutes or until potato topping is golden.

Shepherd's Pie

<u>Ingredients</u>

- 2 teaspoons oil
- 500g lean beef mince
- 1 cup canned, pureed tomatoes, well drained
- 1 cup vegetables, diced (for example, capsicum, carrot, zucchini)
- 3 potatoes
- 2 tablespoons margarine
- ½ cup low fat cheese, grated, reserve some for the top

<u>Method</u>

Preheat oven to 180°C.

Cook beef until brown and add the tomatoes and vegetables and simmer until mixture reduces and thickens. Transfer to a baking dish.

To make topping, cook the potatoes, add margarine and cheese (reserve some cheese for the top) and mash. Add to the beef mixture and sprinkle with the reserved cheese. Bake for 15 minutes.

"Honey Soy" Chicken

Ingredients

- 1 cup zucchini, sliced
- 3 carrots, cut into matchsticks
- 600g chicken breast, cut into strips
- 3 tablespoons rice syrup
- 2 tablespoons wheat free tamari
- 50g walnut halves

Method

Steam the carrots and the zucchini until tender and set aside.

Brown the chicken in a non-stick pan using oil spray. Add the rice syrup and tamari sauce to the chicken and stir in the carrots and zucchini. Cook for 2 minutes. Add the walnuts and serve.

Beef Casserole

Ingredients

- 2 tablespoons oil
- 2 tablespoons margarine
- 2 large carrots, sliced
- 500g beef, chopped into 2.5cm cubes
- 1 large potato, cut into 2cm cubes
- 2 tablespoons gluten free plain flour
- 2 tablespoons wheat free soy sauce
- ½ cup dry red wine
- 1 cup prepared, onion and garlic free, beef stock
- 200g can chopped tomatoes, well drained

Method

Heat half the oil and half the margarine and cook the beef on high heat for 2 minutes, or until browned. Transfer the beef and juices to a bowl.

Heat the remaining oil and add the potato and carrots and cook on medium heat, stirring, for 3 – 5 minutes. Add the flour, wheat free soy sauce and margarine and cook on medium heat, stirring for 1 minute. Turn up the heat to high and add the beef and juices and wine, cook stirring, for 2 minutes or until wine has reduced by half. Return heat to medium-low, add stock and tomatoes and simmer uncovered for 1 ½ to 1 ¾ hours, stirring occasionally until beef is tender and sauce is thick. Serves 4

Tuna Pasta Mornay

Ingredients

- 250g pkt of gluten free penne or spiral pasta
- 425g can tuna, drained
- 1 ½ cups reduced fat cheese, grated
- 1 cup lactose free milk or rice milk
- 1 ½ cups Liddells™ Lactose Free, Light Cream
- 1 cup vegetables, diced (for example, carrots, zucchini, capsicum)
- ½ cup gluten free breadcrumbs and low fat, grated cheese for topping (optional)

Method

Preheat oven to 180°C.

In a saucepan cook the pasta until just tender, drain and run under cold water to stop the cooking process. Set aside.

In another saucepan cook the vegetables for 4 – 5 minutes. Add the cream and milk and simmer, stirring, for 2 – 3 minutes. Stir in the pasta, tuna and cheese. Transfer to an oven proof baking dish, sprinkle with the combined breadcrumbs and cheese and bake until brown.

Serves 4

Alfredo

Ingredients

- ¼ cup low fat margarine
- ½ cup rice milk or lactose free milk
- 1 cup Liddells™ Lactose free, low fat cream
- 1 cup low fat cheese, grated
- 250g gluten free fettuccine
- Sprinkle of parmesan cheese

Method

Whilst boiling pasta, melt margarine in a large pan and add cream, bringing to the boil. Simmer for 5 minutes, stirring constantly. Add the cheese and ½ cup of milk and season well. Reduce heat, add drained pasta and toss until coated. Sprinkle with parmesan.

Macadamia Cookies

Ingredients

- 70g macadamia nuts, finely chopped
- 5 macadamia nuts, halved
- 30g margarine, melted
- ¼ cup of icing sugar
- ½ teaspoon vanilla essence
- ½ cup gluten free plain flour

Method

Preheat oven to 180°C. Line an oven tray with baking paper.

Mix together the margarine, sifted icing sugar and vanilla until light and fluffy, add finely chopped nuts and stir into the flour.

Shape a teaspoon of the mixture into 10 balls and place onto oven tray at least 3cm apart. Press a half macadamia nut into each ball and bake for approximately 10 minutes or until golden brown.

Makes 10 biscuits

Cornflake Cookies

<u>Ingredients</u>

- 100g low fat margarine
- 1 ½ cups gluten free cornflakes
- 1 ½ cups gluten free plain flour
- ¼ cup lactose free milk or rice milk
- 1 teaspoon baking powder

<u>Method</u>

Preheat oven to 180°C. Line an oven tray with baking paper.

Use an electric mixer to combine the margarine and sugar until creamy. Add the flour, baking powder and milk and mix on low speed until a dough is formed.

Stir in the cornflakes with a wooden spoon until combined (cornflakes will crush). Place tablespoons of mixture on the baking tray and slightly flatten with the back of a spoon.

Bake for 10 – 15 minutes until golden.

Muesli Bars

Ingredients

- ½ cup gluten free plain flour
- ½ cup rice syrup (warmed to mix easier)
- 2 tablespoons low fat margarine, melted
- 3 cups Food for Health™ Clusters muesli
- 2 eggs, lightly whisked

Method

Preheat oven to 180°C. Line a lamington tray with baking paper.

Mix muesli and flour. Add eggs, warmed rice syrup and margarine.

Mix thoroughly until all combined and sticky.

Press mixture into the prepared lamington tray and bake for 30

minutes. Cut muesli into slices whilst still warm and allow to cool

in tray.

Macadamia Brittle

Ingredients

- 1 cup macadamia nuts
- 1 cup caster sugar
- ¼ cup water
- 1 heaped tablespoon low fat margarine

Method

Line a small baking tray with alfoil.

Place the nuts evenly on the tray.

Boil the water and sugar until mixture turns golden. Add the margarine, stir (mixture will bubble and froth) and quickly pour over the nuts.

Allow to cool to set and break into serves.

CAKES

Vanilla Cake

Makes one large cake or 12 muffins

Ingredients

- ½ cup caster sugar
- 170g margarine
- 3 eggs
- 100ml lactose free milk or rice milk
- 1 ½ cup gluten free self raising flour
- 1/3 cup cornflour

Method

Preheat oven to 180°C or 160°C for a fan-forced oven.

Using an electric mixer, mix the caster sugar, margarine, 3 eggs and milk until well combined. Add the flours and beat for 2 to 3 minutes.

Bake for 30 minutes for a large cake or 20 minutes for 12 muffins [or until a toothpick comes out clean].

Banana Cake

Ingredients

- ½ cup margarine, softened
- ½ cup castor sugar
- 2 eggs
- 1 teaspoon bicarbonate soda
- ½ cup lactose free milk or rice milk
- 2 large bananas, mashed
- 2 cups gluten free self raising flour

Method

Pre-heat oven to 180°C. Lightly grease a loaf tin. In a large mixing bowl cream the margarine and sugar. Add the eggs one at a time, beating well after each addition.

In a separate bowl, combine the bicarbonate soda and milk, add the bananas and add this mixture to the egg mixture and beat until well combined. Fold in the flour and stir until just combined.

Spoon into the prepared tin and bake for 45 to 50 minutes or until cooked when tested with a skewer. Cool in tin for 5 minutes and turn onto a wire rack to cool completely.

Strawberry or Blueberry Rice Cake

Ingredients

- 3 cups lactose free milk or rice milk
- 1 cup short-grain rice
- ¼ cup firmly packed brown sugar
- 60g low fat margarine, melted
- 2 eggs, lightly beaten
- 150g frozen blueberries or strawberries

Method

Preheat oven to 180°C. Lightly grease a loaf tin or round cake tin.
In a saucepan, bring the milk and rice slowly to the boil. Reduce
heat, cover and simmer, stirring occasionally, for 30 minutes or
until rice is soft. Add the sugar and margarine and mix well. Set
aside to cool.

When cool, add the beaten eggs to the rice mixture and combine.
Spoon half this mixture into the prepared tin, add the blueberries
or strawberries, then top with the remaining mixture.

Bake for 40 minutes or until top is golden brown and has formed a
crust. Transfer to a rack to cool slightly before serving.

DESSERTS

Rhubarb / Strawberry Soufflé

Ingredients

- ½ bunch rhubarb stalks, chopped
- 1 cup frozen or fresh strawberries (thawed), chopped
- 4 egg whites
- 2 tablespoons brown sugar
- ¼ cup caster sugar

Method

Preheat oven to 180°C. Lightly grease four 1-cup capacity ramekins. Combine the rhubarb, brown sugar and 2 tablespoons of water in a saucepan, bring to the boil, reduce heat and simmer for 5 minutes until rhubarb tender. Add the strawberries and simmer for a further 2 minutes. Divide the mixture between the ramekins. Using an electric beater, beat the egg whites until soft peaks form. Add the caster sugar, one tablespoon at a time, beating well after each addition until sugar is dissolved. Spoon over the fruit mixture. Bake for 8 – 12 minutes or until browned and puffed.

Serves 4

Pavlova

Ingredients

- 4 large egg whites
- 150g caster sugar
- 1 teaspoon cream of tartar
- 200g tub Liddells™ Lactose Free, Plain Yoghurt
- Allowable fruit for topping

Method

Preheat oven to 110°C. Line a baking tray with non-stick baking paper.

In a large bowl, beat the eggs with an electric hand whisk on medium speed until stiff peaks form.

Beat in the caster sugar, one spoon at a time, on high speed. Continue to whisk until the mixture is stiff and glossy. Add the cream of tartar and whisk until well combined.

Transfer the egg white mixture to the prepared baking tray creating an approximate 20cm diameter round shape.

Bake for 2 hours. Turn the oven off and allow the pavlova to cool inside the oven until the oven is completely cold.

Top with fruit and yoghurt immediately prior to serving.

Lemon Dessert

Ingredients

- 20g low fat margarine
- 2 eggs, separated
- 1 tablespoon caster sugar
- 1 tablespoon lemon juice
- 1 teaspoon finely grated lemon rind
- ½ cup lactose free milk or rice milk
- 1 tablespoon gluten free self raising flour

Method

Preheat oven to 180°C. Lightly grease three ramekins or teacups. Beat the sugar, margarine and lemon rind until light and creamy. Beat in the egg yolks and lemon juice. Fold in the flour and milk. Beat the egg whites until soft peaks form and fold into the lemon mixture. The mixture will remain slightly lumpy. Divide between the 3 ramekins or teacups. Place into a deep baking dish and fill dish with enough water to come half way up the sides of the ramekins and bake for 45 minutes.

Serves 3

Strawberry Ice Cream

Ingredients

- 1 cup frozen strawberries
- ½ cup icing sugar
- ½ cup Liddells™ Lactose Free, Plain Yoghurt

Method

Process the frozen berries in a processor, add the icing sugar and the yoghurt and process to combine.

Serve in chilled dishes.

Vanilla Risotto

Ingredients

- 900ml lactose free milk
- 160g Arborio rice
- 60g sugar
- 1 ½ teaspoons vanilla extract

Method

Place milk and rice into a saucepan and cook until rice softens. Add the sugar and vanilla and leave for 10 minutes to cool and thicken. Serve

Vanilla Quinoa Pudding

Ingredients

- ½ cup quinoa, rinsed and drained
- 2 large eggs
- ¼ teaspoon ground cinnamon
- ¼ cup sugar
- 3 cups lactose free milk or rice milk
- 1 teaspoon vanilla essence

Method

In a large saucepan add quinoa and milk and bring to the boil. Reduce heat to low and simmer, stirring occasionally, for approximately 15 minutes or until soft.

In a small mixing bowl, whisk together the eggs, cinnamon, sugar and vanilla and slowly add the mixture to the quinoa whilst stirring over heat. Cook for a further 5 minutes, or until thickened. Pour into 6 serving dishes, cover and refrigerate for at least 2 hours before serving.

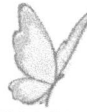

Bibliography

American College of Gastroenterology IBS Task Force. An evidence-based position statement on the management of irritable bowel syndrome. Am. J. Gastroenterology 2009;104:S1-S35.

Barrett JS, Gibson PR. Clinical ramifications of malabsorption of fructose and other short-chain carbohydrates. *Pract. Gastroenterol.* 2007; 51-65

Biesiekierski JR, Rosella O, Rose R, et al. Quantification of fructans, galacto-oligosaccharides and other short-chain carbohydrates in processed grains and cereals. J Hum Nutr Diet 2011;24:154-176.

Bijkerk CJ, Muris JW, Knottnerus JA, Hoes AW, de Wit NJ. Systematic review: The role of different types of fibre in the treatment of irritable bowel syndrome. Aliment. Pharmacol. Ther. 2004;19:245-251.

Department of Gastroenterology & Department of Nutrition and Dietetics Guy's and St Thomas' NHS Foundation Trust and King's College London: Reintroducing FODMAPs. January 2011. www.kcl.ac.uk/fodmaps

Floch MH, Narayan R. Diet in the irritable bowel syndrome. J. Clin. Gastroenterol. 2002;35(Suppl.):S45-S52.

Gibson PR, Shepherd SJ. Evidence-based dietary management of functional gastrointestinal symptoms: The FODMAP approach. J. Gastroenterol. Hepatol. 2010; 252-258

Gonzalez R, Dunkel R, Koletzko B, Schusdziarra V, Allescher HD. Effect of capsaicin-containing red pepper sauce suspension on upper gastrointestinal motility in healthy volunteers. Digestive Diseases and Sciences 1998;43:1165-1171

Hammer J, Hammer K, Kletter K. Lipids infused into the jejunum accelerate small intestinal transit but delay ileocolonic transit of solids and liquids. Gut 1998; 43:111-116.

Heizer WD, Southern S, McGovern S. The role of diet in symptoms of irritable bowel syndrome in adults: A narrative review. J. Am. Diet. Assoc. 2009;109:1204-1214.

Li BW, Andrews KW, Pehrsson PR. Individual sugars, soluble and insoluble dietary fibre contents of 70 high consumption foods. J. Food Comp. Anal. 2002;15:715-723.

Mayer EA, Naliboff BD, Chang L, Coutinho SV. Stress and the gastrointestinal tract v. stress and irritable bowel syndrome. Am J Physiol. Gastrointest. Liver Physiol. 2001;280:G519-G524.

Monash University. The low FODMAP diet. 2010
http://www.med.monash.edu.au/ehcs.

Muir JG, Rose R, Rosella O, Liels K, Barrett JS, Shepherd SJ, Gibson PR. Measurement of short-chain carbohydrates in common Australian vegetables and fruits by high-performance liquid chromatography (HPLC). J. Agric. Food Chem., 2009; 57:554-565

Muir JG, Shepherd SJ, Rosella O, Rose R, Gibson PR. Fructan and free fructose content of common Australian fruit and vegetables. J. Arigc. Food Chem. 2007;55:6619-6627

Nobaek S, Johansson ML, Molin G, Ahrne S, Jeppson B. Alteration of intestinal microflora is associated with reduction in abdominal bloating and pain in patients with irritable bowel syndrome. Am. J. Gastroenterol. 2000 May;95(5):1231-8.

Rao SS, Welcher K, Zimmerman B, Stumbo P. Is coffee a colonic stimulant? Eur. J. Gastroenterol. Hepatol. 1998;10:113-118.

Shepherd SJ, Gibson PR. Fructose malabsorption and symptoms of irritable bowel syndrome: guidelines for effective dietary management. J AM Diet Assoc. 2006;106:1631-1639

Simren M, Abrahamsson H, Bjornsson ES. An exaggerated sensory component of the gastrocolonic response in patients with irritable bowel syndrome. Gut 2001; 48:20-27.

Simren M, Mansson A, Langkilde AM, Svedlund J, Abrahamsson H, Bengtsson U, Bjornsson ES. Food-related gastrointestinal symptoms in the irritable bowel syndrome. Digestion 2001;63:108-115.